Understanding GOUT

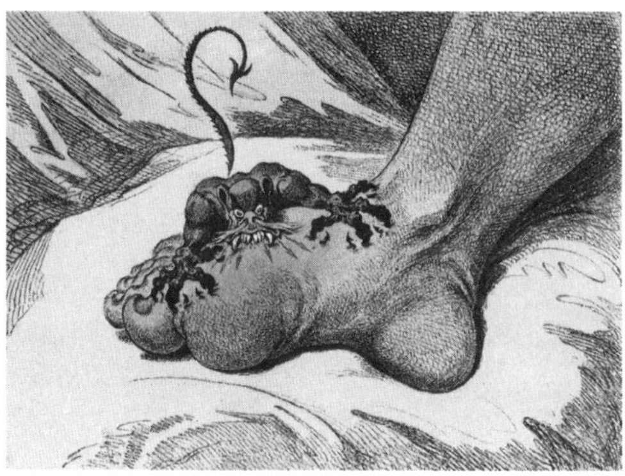

Warren Jefferson

live healthy now!

HEALTHY LIVING PUBLICATIONS
Summertown, Tennessee

Cover and interior design: Scattaregia Design

Healthy Living Publications,
a division of Book Publishing Company
P.O. Box 99
Summertown, TN 38483
888-260-8458
www.bookpubco.com

ISBN: 978-1-57067-298-9

Printed in The United States of America

19 18 17 16 15 14 1 2 3 4 5 6 7 8 9

Library of Congress Cataloging-in-Publication Data

Jefferson, Warren, 1943-
Understanding gout / Warren Jefferson.
pages cm
Includes bibliographical references.
ISBN 978-1-57067-298-9 (pbk.) -- ISBN 978-1-57067-889-9 (e-book)
1. Gout--Popular works. I. Title.
RC629.J44 2014
616.3'999--dc23
2014018181

Printed on recycled paper

Book Publishing Company is a member of Green Press Initiative. We chose to print this title on paper with 100% post consumer recycled content, processed without chlorine, which saved the following natural resources:

- 18 trees
- 563 pounds of solid waste
- 8,414 gallons of water
- 1,551 pounds of greenhouse gases
- 8 million BTU of energy

For more information on Green Press Initiative, visit www.greenpressinitiative.org. Environmental impact estimates were made using the Environmental Defense Fund Paper Calculator. For more information visit www.papercalculator.org.

CONTENTS

PREFACE

With this book I have attempted to give gout sufferers and the people who love them a comprehensive view of the disease—the latest recommendations on diet and lifestyle, both modern and ancient treatments, natural remedies, and the history of gout, the disease Hippocrates (400 BCE) called *podagra*, the unwalkable disease.

In doing the research for this book I have drawn from the following sources among others:

American College of Physicians
American College of Rheumatology
3E Recommendations in Rheumatology
The Cleveland Clinic Journal of Medicine
The Mayo Clinic
National Institute of Arthritis and Musculoskeletal and Skin Diseases
The National Institute of Health
New York University Hospital for Joint Disease
The University of Maryland Medical Center

I have also referenced a number of leading rheumatologists and experts on gout. I want to thank David Goldfarb, MD, Francis Roubille, MD, and Robert Kennan, MD, for their critical review of the manuscript.

INTRODUCTION

Thomas Sydenham, the "English Hippocrates" of the seventeenth century and himself a gout sufferer, once stated, "Great kings, emperors, generals, admirals, and philosophers have all died of gout. Hereby Nature shows her impartiality, since those whom she favors in one way she afflicts in another—a mixture of good and evil pre-eminently adapted to our frail mortality."

Gout is as significant a disease today as it was when first described by the Greek physician Aretaeus of Cappadocia in the first century CE. It has been the bane of humanity long before the beginning of western medicine. The Egyptians knew about the disease as early as 2640 BCE.

Gout was historically referred to as "the disease of kings," because it was associated with a diet of rich foods (such as organ meats and sweets) and the consumption of immoderate amounts of alcohol, particularly ale. Cicero, King Henry VII, Francis Bacon, Michelangelo, Peter Paul Rubens, Galileo Galilei, Sir Isaac Newton, Ben Franklin, and Charles Darwin all suffered from its debilitating effects. It was such a prominent part of life in the 17th and 18th centuries that people afflicted with gout would refer to their condition as having "The Gout."

Fortunately, people no longer die of gout, but it's still a significant disease and one that's often misdiagnosed and treated improperly. The average person in a developed country now eats as well as a king, so gout is also afflicting them, not just the wealthy. Reported cases of gout are increasing worldwide, having doubled in the United States in the last twenty years.

Currently, much is known about gout—its progression, symptoms, and risk factors; how to treat it; and what causes an acute gout flare—but little is known about the underlying cause of the disease and why some people with specific preconditions for gout develop symptoms and others do not.

It's been long suspected that a diet containing a high level of animal protein foods was a causal factor in the development of hyperuricemia and gout, and a study published in the *New England Journal of Medicine* has confirmed this. High-fructose corn syrup also has been shown to have a direct effect on gout symptoms. It's generally recommended that gout patients reduce the consumption of all types of sugar, including fructose. Alcohol consumption—especially beer—has been shown to increase uric acid production and inhibit its elimination. (Wine in moderation does not have this same effect.)

If left untreated, gout can have serious health effects. Between 1965 and 2009 there had been virtually no research on gout and no new drugs developed for treating it. Since the beginning of the twenty-first century there's been renewed interest, and the development of treatments for gout is advancing once again. A new generation of researchers has begun looking at the underlying processes of hyperuricemia and how it leads to gout. We now have new drugs and biological agents on the market (as well as others under development) that are giving doctors more options for treating gout.

If someone is diagnosed as having gout and has had a gout flare, they will most likely have further flares. They'll have to take urate-lowering medications for some years, maybe for the rest of their life. Although we don't know the exact cause of gout and gout can't really be cured, even with proper treatment, it can be effectively managed and controlled. Uric acid levels can return to normal, crystal buildup stopped, gout flares reduced or eliminated, and disfiguring deposits dissolved. Gout sufferers need not be sufferers anymore and can lead normal lives free of gout's debilitating effects.

What Is Gout?

Gout is a type of arthritis, a chronic, degenerative disease of the joints and one of the most common inflammatory arthritic conditions. A gout attack or flare is one of the most painful, acute medical conditions a person can experience. Gout is often called a man's disease, because the vast majority of sufferers are men in the prime of life. It affects up to one to two percent of men in Western countries and approximately 3.4 million American men. Postmenopausal women can also be affected, but to a lesser degree, and they make up only about five percent of the total cases in the United States. Although the prevalence is greater in men, the rate of incidence in women comes close to reaching that of men by the time they reach age seventy-five to eighty.

It appears that people can have a genetic predisposition to developing gout. As John Hardin, chairman of the Department of Medicine at Albert Einstein College of Medicine describes it, "gout is 90 percent a disease of genetics and 10 percent a disease of lifestyle, and until we can target the genes responsible, gout will remain an incurable disease."

Gout is characterized by spontaneous episodes of inflammation and intense pain to one or more joints. It's also a crystal arthritis disease (joint inflammation caused by crystal deposits) and considered a rheumatic disease. (In the medical literature, the terms arthritis and rheumatism are used interchangeably.) Additionally, it's a metabolic disorder because it disrupts chemical processes that occur within the body.

Gout is associated with a metabolic condition called hyperuricemia, in which there is a supersaturation of uric acid (a natural by-product of metabolism) in a person's blood plasma. In some people, hyperuricemia can lead to the deposit of monosodium urate crystals in joints and soft tissue. When crystal buildup reaches a critical point, the crystals can shed or be released into the synovial fluid in the joint. This causes a sudden gout flare with inflammation, swelling, and intense pain. In a large majority of cases, the initial location is the first joint of the big toe, and the flare-up usually occurs in the middle of the night or early morning.

You normally generate between 250 and 750 milligrams of uric acid a day from body cell turnover and the foods you eat. Normally uric acid is dissolved in the blood and most is passed through the kidneys into the urine and eliminated. A small percentage is processed through the digestive tract.

However, if there's an increase in the production of uric acid or the kidneys don't eliminate enough uric acid (or both), urate builds up in the blood, joint fluids, and tissue, causing hyperuricemia. In 10 to 15 percent of gout sufferers, hyperuricemia is the result of overproduction of uric acid; in 85 to 90 percent, it's the result of renal impairment or underexcretion by the kidneys (or a combination of the two). The normal blood level of urate is from 4 to 6.8 mg/dL. A level greater than 7 mg/dL is considered hyperuricemia.

In people with a predisposition for gout, persistent hyperuricemia leads to the depositing of monosodium urate (MSU) crystals in joints and surrounding tissue. MSU crystals can also form in the kidneys (as kidney stones) and other organs. If gout is left untreated, this crystal deposition will cause chronic, acute inflammation, leading over time to joint destruction, deformity, and other complications.

Stages of Gout

The progression of gout follows four stages:

1. Asymptomatic hyperuricemia
2. Acute gout (acute gouty arthritis)
3. Interval or intercritical gout
4. Chronic tophaceous gout

Asymptomatic Hyperuricemia

Currently there's no reliable way to predict that a particular person with asymptomatic hyperuricemia (without symptoms) will develop gout. In fact, less than 20 percent of people who are asymptomatic end up with gout. As a result, asymptomatic hyperuricemia is currently not considered a disease. Treatment at this stage is generally not recommended unless a person has a strong family history of gout, is about to receive chemotherapy, has a history of kidney stones, has moderate renal impairment, is a binge alcohol drinker, or has a uric level of at least 12 or 13 mg/dL in men and 10 mg/dL in women.

The progression from asymptomatic hyperuricemia to chronic gout can be quite variable and take anywhere from ten to thirty years. During this time, levels of urate in the blood can reach 7 mg/dL or higher, and although MSU crystals are accumulating, no other symptoms may appear. However, individuals with this condition are at increased risk for metabolic syndrome (obesity, high blood pressure, elevated cholesterol, and high blood sugar) and cardiovascular disease and should be screened for these conditions. Also, they should be informed about the importance of healthy lifestyle factors, such as a nutritious diet and regular exercise.

Acute Gout (Acute Gouty Arthritis)

Acute gout occurs with the initial onset of symptoms. By this stage, hyperuricemia has caused critical amounts of MSU crystals to deposit in one or more joints. Eventually these crystals shed from the joint cartilage and become mobilized in the joint space. This leads to an auto-inflammatory response and the joint becomes swollen and inflamed. The skin over the joint becomes red, shiny, and tight, and may peel after a few days. The affected joint is impaired and very sensitive to the touch. If a joint in the lower extremities is involved, walking is difficult if not impossible.

Acute gout attacks or flares can include low-grade fever, chills, loss of appetite, and malaise. Over time, attacks can last longer and occur more frequently. A gout flare consists of several painful episodes and commonly occurs at night or early morning. A flare can be triggered by trauma to a joint, a stressful event, binge drinking, drugs, or the presence of another illness.

Untreated symptoms reach a peak in twelve to twenty-four hours after onset. A gout flare is self-limiting, in that symptoms ultimately subside in one to two weeks and the person can return to normal activities. Medical experts aren't sure what brings on a remission.

Sixty percent of first-time gout flares among middle-aged adults occur only in one joint (monoarticular). The primary location is usually the first joint of the big toe (podagra), but other joints and tissues around the joints can be affected. Ten to twenty percent of first attacks occur in multiple joints (polyarticular), including the insteps, ankles, heels, knees, wrists, fingers, and elbows. Older people tend to develop polyarticular gout.

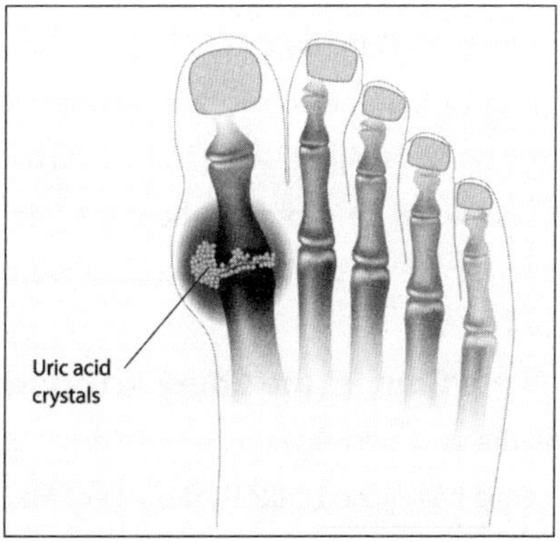

Gout usually affects joints in the toes or fingers first, since blood temperature decreases the further from the heart that circulation occurs. MSU crystals form at normal body temperature when the urate level in the blood reaches the saturation point of 7 mg/dL. However, at lower temperatures, crystals can form at a urate level below 7 mg/dL.

The following is a first-person account of an acute gout attack suffered by the English physician, Thomas Sydenham whose quote starts off this book's introduction:

> Towards the end of January or the beginning of February suddenly, and with scarcely any premonitory feelings, the disease breaks out. Its only forerunner is indigestion and crudity of the stomach, which troubles the patient for some weeks previous to the attack. His body also feels swollen, heavy, and windy—symptoms which increase from day to day until the fit breaks out. But a few days before this torpor comes on, sic [there is] a feeling of flatus along the legs and thighs. Besides this there is spasmodic affection, whilst the day before the fit the appetite is unnaturally hearty.
>
> The victim goes to bed in good health and sleeps. About two o'clock in the morning he is awakened by a severe pain,

generally in the great toe, more rarely in the heel, ankle, or instep. This pain is like that of a dislocation of the bones of these parts, and is accompanied by a sensation as of chilly water poured over the membranes of the suffering joint.

Then follows chills and shivers and a little fever. The pain, which was at first moderate, becomes gradually more intense, and while it increases, the chills and shivers die out. Every hour that passes finds it greater, until at length at night-time it reaches its worst intensity, and insinuates itself with most exquisite cruelty among the numerous small bones of the tarsus and metatarsus, in the ligament of which it is lurking. Now it is a violent stretching and tearing of the ligaments—now it is a gnawing pain and now a pressure and tightening. So exquisite and lively meanwhile is the feeling of the part affected, that it cannot bear the weight of bedclothes nor the jar of a person walking in the room.

Hence the night is passed in torture, and a restless rolling first to one side, then to the other, of the suffering limb, with perpetual change of posture, the tossing about of the body being as incessant as the pain of the tortured joint, and being at its worst as the fit is coming on. Hence the vain efforts by change of posture, both in the body and the limb affected, to obtain an abatement of the pain.

Interval or Intercritical Gout

Intercritical gout is the period between acute gout attacks. In this stage, a gout sufferer doesn't have clinical symptoms, but MSU crystal buildup continues to occur. Left untreated, gout flares return in most cases. More than two-thirds of people will have a second gout attack within two years, and by ten years, 90 percent of them will have repeat attacks.

Chronic Tophaceous Gout

Persistent hyperuricemia can lead to chronic tophaceous gout, a condition that includes the formation of solid deposits of MSU crystals known as *tophi.* Tophi form as lumps under the skin and in joints, cartilage, bones, and elsewhere in the body. They can break through the skin and appear as white or yellowish-white nodules. Tophi are usually painless during formation.

This stage usually develops over a long period of time, typically ten years, but can range from three to forty-two years after the initial onset of gout. Tophi can grow to the size of golf balls and if left untreated can lead to bone erosion and cartilage damage.

Tophi can form in any of these locations:

- along the ridge of the outer ear
- forearms
- elbow or knee
- hands or feet
- around the vocal cords, heart, and spine (rarely)

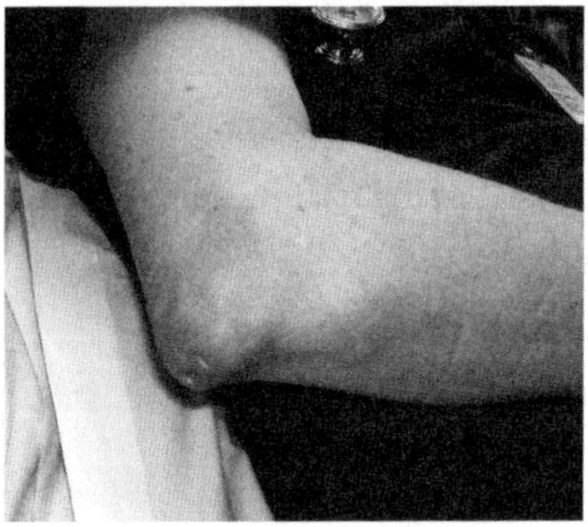

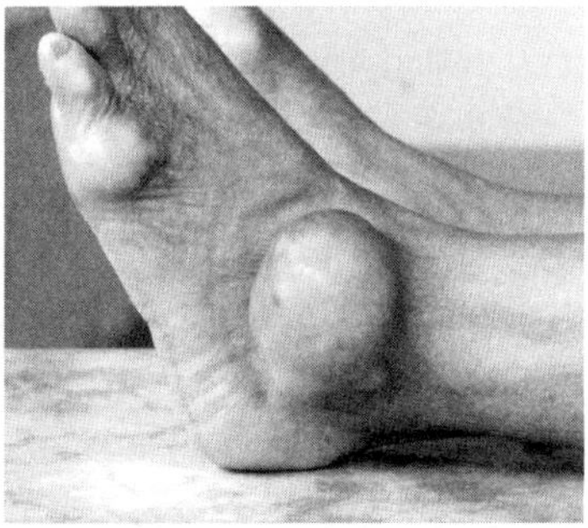

Tophi formation and discomfort have been documented since ancient times. Aretaeus, writing in the second century AD, made the following observations concerning tophi: "Callosities also form in the joints; at first they resemble abscesses, but afterwards they get more condensed, and the humour being condensed is difficult to dissolve; at last they are converted into hard white tophi."

Sir Alfred Baring Garrod (1857–1936), discussing tophi on the fingers of one of his patients, said they looked like "small, rounded protuberances" with the skin being red. When he punctured one of them, "a thin, white fluid exuded." When he placed a drop under a microscope in polarized light, he could see crystals that upon analysis consisted of urate of soda.

British physician L. J. Llewellyn, in his 1921 tome simply titled *Gout*, writes that: "Tophi are always preceded by local inflammatory reactions of varying grades of severity, and that the uratic deposits are sequels thereto. In their early stages their presence is betokened by soft red swellings associated with sensations of pricking and tenderness. Their transmutation into white pearly concretions is a process that takes months to mature."

In the elderly, tophi may appear earlier than ten years after the onset of gout. Elderly women are at higher risk for developing tophi than middle-aged men with gout, and they usually develop tophi in the finger joints.

This is the most disabling stage of gout and carries the risk of permanent damage to the affected joints. Sometimes the kidneys and other organs can also be affected. But with the use of urate-lowering therapy (ULT), most patients don't progress to this advanced stage. MSU crystal buildup can be stopped, the body cleared of crystals, and tophi dissolved and eliminated.

Understanding Uric Acid

Uric acid is the relatively insoluble end product of the metabolism of a substance called purine. Purines are an integral part of cell function. They're found in the cells of all animals and plants and are part of the chemical structure of DNA and RNA, the genetic material of all cells. Purines are produced when these genetic materials are metabolized. Purines formed by bodily processes account for 70 percent of the amount in your body, while 30 percent are derived from diet.

Although too much uric acid or urate in the blood can be problem, uric acid is an important antioxidant and helps to protect blood vessel linings and other tissues. A consistent supply of uric acid circulating in the body is essential for maintaining health.

Some foods have a high concentration of purines. For the most part, these are high-protein foods such as animal meats (beef, pork, lamb, organ meats, and meat extracts), seafood (mackerel, herring, sardines, tuna, shrimp, lobster, clams, mussels, etc.), and some plant foods (yeast extracts, peas, beans, lentils, asparagus, and mushrooms). Low-purine foods include dairy products, grains, most vegetables, fruits, sugars, and sweets.

Purines present somewhat of a mystery. We know that some foods contain high amounts of purines and others do not, but we don't know a lot about the identity and quantity of the purines in most foods. We know even less about purines in cooked and processed foods. See "A Recommended Diet for Chronic Gout," page 30, for more information.

Recent research in genetic anthropology has indicated that uric acid may have played an important role in human evolution and survival. Most mammals have a urate level below 2 mg/dL, but humans have urate levels of 4 to 7 mg/dL.

Nephrologist Richard Johnson, a professor at the University of Colorado in Denver, has a theory as to why our urate levels are so much higher. He speculates that some 10 to 22 million years ago humans lost the ability to synthesize uricase, a compound that breaks down uric acid into a more easily excreted compound, allantonin. During that period, the primate diet was vegetarian for the most part and consisted of fruits and grasses that were low in sodium. Hyperuricemia is known to raise blood pressure (hyperuricemia is associated with hypertension), and the theory goes that the loss of uricase and the ability to process uric acid was an evolutionary adaptation by primates to maintain or raise blood pressure sufficiently to allow blood to reach the brain during upright walking.

Johnson also believes that since uric acid inhibits an enzyme that breaks down fat, a lack of uricase could have provided an adaptive advantage against starvation by allowing increased storage of body fat. However, overabundance and excess fat storage, not starvation, are major contributors to health problems in developed nations today, so that adaptation is now a detriment.

Your Risk for Gout

A person is more likely to develop gout if he or she has one or more of the following risk factors.

Hyperuricemia

The vast majority of people with gout have hyperuricemia, so hyperuricemia is considered the major risk factor for gout.

Gender and Age

When men reach puberty, their uric acid levels increase significantly. For this reason, men are at a significantly higher risk for developing gout than women. The risk for gout also goes up with increasing age. In people under the age of 45, the prevalence is 1.8 in 1,000 people. In people over 65, it jumps to 30.8 in 1,000 people!

As was stated earlier, it takes from ten to thirty years of persistent hyperuricemia and MSU crystal buildup for a gout flare to occur. Men who are susceptible to gout usually experience their first attack in middle age, but some people experience gout much earlier, in their twenties or thirties.

After menopause, women too are at an increased risk for gout. The lower risk factor before menopause is attributed to higher estrogen levels. Estrogen helps uric acid elimination. After age sixty, women make up approximately half the new cases of gout. At age eighty, the rate of gout in women is higher than in men. Gout is rare in children unless there is an inherited genetic defect causing hyperuricemia.

Family History

It's been known for centuries that there's a genetic predisposition to gout. There have been three gene locations identified with the processing of uric acid and purines. People with gout have a defect in these genes that interferes with their ability to metabolize purines and eliminate uric acid through the kidneys.

If someone in your family has gout, you have at least a 20 percent risk of developing the disease. Interestingly, in many families with a history of gout, the disease may skip a generation. If your father didn't have gout, you may still be at risk if your grandfather did.

Diet

Consuming purine-rich foods, such as meat and certain seafood, raises the level of uric acid in the body and increases the risk for gout and acute gout attacks. Most rheumatologists recommend giving up or greatly reducing the consumption of meat and seafood.

Fructose is the only carbohydrate known to increase uric acid levels. According to a study reported in the *British Medical Journal* in 2008, "prospective data suggest that consumption of sugar-sweetened soft drinks and fructose is strongly associated with an increased risk of gout in men. Furthermore, fructose-rich fruits and fruit juices may also increase the risk. Diet soft drinks were not associated with the risk of gout." See page 31 for more information.

Alcohol Consumption

High alcohol intake, especially beer (which is rich in the readily absorbed purine guanosine) and to a lesser extent spirits, has been shown to increase uric acid production and inhibit its elimination. Consumption of these beverages constitutes a risk factor for gout flares and should be avoided. Wine on the other hand has been shown to contribute no negative effects if consumed in moderation: two five-ounce drinks per day for men (one for women), according to the Mayo Clinic.

Obesity

Obesity greatly increases risk for hyperuricemia and gout. Extra fat in the torso, as measured by body mass index (BMI) and waist-to-hip ratio, can be a predictor for gout. A Japanese study showed that overweight people had two to three times the rate of hyperuricemia as people with a healthy weight. In a comparison of men with a near-ideal weight (BMI of 25), overweight men (BMI of 25 to 29.9) have almost double the risk of developing gout, and the risk is nearly tripled for those with a BMI of 35 or greater.

Medical Conditions

A number of medical situations can elevate risk for gout. Some of these are particular medical conditions, while others can range from treatments and medications to lifestyle and environmental factors, and even organ transplantation.

A large percentage of people with gout have metabolic syndrome (MetS), which is becoming a major medical problem in the United States. MetS is a group of medical conditions that can occur together and include

Risk Factors for Gout

- high uric acid levels, hyperuricemia
- male
- female past menopause
- middle aged or older
- family member had the disease
- diet contains foods high in purines
- consumes fructose
- abuses alcohol
- obese
- various medical conditions, treatments, medications, and lifestyle habits

insulin resistance, pre-diabetes, high cholesterol, hypertension, and abdominal obesity. If a person has three or more of these conditions, they have MetS and are at an increased risk for diabetes and cardiovascular disease (CVD). People with hyperuricemia and gout are at an increased risk for MetS, and having MetS can increase risk for gout as well.

Other medical conditions that are associated with hyperuricemia and gout are peripheral vascular disease (poor circulation in the limbs), hyperlipidemia (fats in the bloodstream), hypothyroidism (underactive thyroid gland), hemolytic anemia, some cancers, psoriasis, and kidney disease. Renal insufficiency, or the inability of the kidneys to eliminate waste products, is a common cause of gout in older people. Kelley-Seegmiller syndrome or Lesch-Nyhan syndrome, two rare conditions in which the enzyme that helps control uric acid levels is lacking, can also cause hyperuricemia. If you have hyperuricemia and also develop osteoarthritic joints, urate crystals are more likely to deposit in those joints.

A number of medications may put people at risk for developing hyperuricemia and gout. The following may increase uric acid and urate:

- Cyclosporine and cyclosporine (modified) used to prevent transplant rejection in patients who've received kidney, liver, and heart transplants and treat rheumatoid arthritis
- Levodopa, a medicine used to support communication along nerve pathways in the treatment of Parkinson's disease
- Niacin, used to treat high cholesterol
- Salicylate-containing drugs, such as aspirin

Diuretics, such as thiazide, which are taken to eliminate excess fluid from the body in conditions like hypertension, edema, and heart disease, decrease the amount of uric acid passed in the urine, thus increasing the amount in the bloodstream.

A 2012 study in the *Annals of Internal Medicine* showed that low-level exposure to lead over time can result in a buildup of uric acid and an increased risk for gout. It's thought that elevated lead levels in the blood can compromise kidney function and lead to an increase in serum urate levels and risk for gout. Chelation therapy can remove lead from the body, resulting in reduced uric acid in the blood.

Other lifestyle habits and situations that can lead to gout are dehydration, fasting, joint injury, and either inactivity or overactivity. Gout patients are advised to drink a minimum of eight cups of water a day in order to encourage urination. Fasting is discouraged, because the level of ketones in the body increases during a fast and competes with uric acid excretion. In people with hyperuricemia, even stubbing the large toe or other joint in the hand or foot can trigger a gout attack.

Diagnosing Gout

No single test can determine if you have gout. The best your doctor can do is perform one or more procedures that can show whether you have high levels of uric acid, urates, MSU crystals, inflammation, or bone erosion.

However, the American College of Rheumatology (ACR) has developed eleven criteria for diagnosis to help doctors identify gout without having to resort to invasive testing. The presence of six or more of these criteria is a strong indication that you have gout:

1. More than one attack of active arthritis
2. Maximum inflammation develops within one day
3. Attack of oligoarthritis (inflammatory arthritis characterized by swelling of only a few joints)
4. Redness observed over a joint
5. Pain or swelling in a first metatarsalophalangeal joint (the large joint of the big toe)
6. Attack in a first metatarsalophalangeal joint
7. Attack in a unilateral tarsal joint (ankle or upper foot)
8. Tophus (proven or suspect)

9. Hyperuricemia (serum uric acid level equal to or greater than 6.8 mg/dL)
10. Asymetrical swelling within a joint on x-rays
11. Complete termination of an attack

Another possible indication of gout is if you have a rapid response to treatment with a drug called colchicine (see page 26).

Some medical conditions can produce gout-like symptoms, and they should be considered before gout can be determined. For instance, there are more than 200 forms of arthritis that can cause joint pain, inflammation, and swelling. Chronic gout is sometimes confused with rheumatoid arthritis, which can distort finger joints and produce inflammation and pain. Calcium pyrophosphate dihydrate crystal deposition disease (CPPD or pseudogout) can also cause deposits in the joints and mimic the symptoms of gout. However, with CPPD these deposits are made up of calcium pyrophosphate, not monosodium urate (MSU).

If there's any doubt as to whether the previous criteria are conclusive, your doctor may prescribe one or more of the following tests.

Synovial Fluid Test

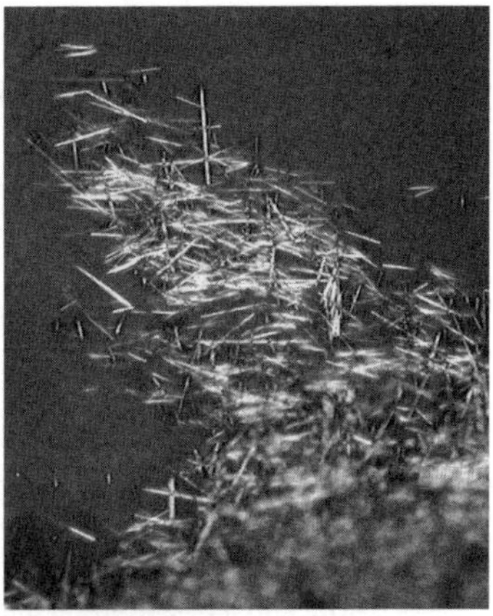

This test, which analyses the lubricating fluid in the joints, is the gold standard of tests for gout. Fluid is taken from the affected joint or tophi with a needle syringe (a procedure called aspiration) and sent to a lab to be examined under a microscope using polarized light to look for the presence of MSU crystals. If crystals are present, so is gout. Aspiration is done without anesthesia because anesthesia can affect the results. The procedure is described as only mildly uncomfortable.

A synovial fluid test can also be used to determine if there might be an infection in the joint (septic arthritis). It can be performed during a gout flare or between flares. This test can also indicate the presence of CPPD.

Urine Test

A twenty-four-hour urine test can show the amount of uric acid in the urine. After the first urination of the day of testing, your doctor will have you collect all the other urine you produce during the following twenty-four hours, including the first urination of the day following. This is done during a period when you have no symptoms and after you've been following a purine-reduced diet for some time.

Serum Uric Acid Test

In a serum uric acid test, a sample of blood is drawn and the amount of uric acid in the blood is measured. A high level of uric acid in the blood is a strong indication of gout but doesn't confirm it conclusively. During urate-lowering therapy, serum uric acid tests are useful for monitoring urate levels.

Radiography

X-rays can't show uric acid buildup in the joints, but it can show the effects of gout, such as bone erosion. It can also help differentiate gout from rheumatoid arthritis and rule out other conditions, like CPPD. X-rays can reveal the presence of tophi before they're apparent in physical examinations.

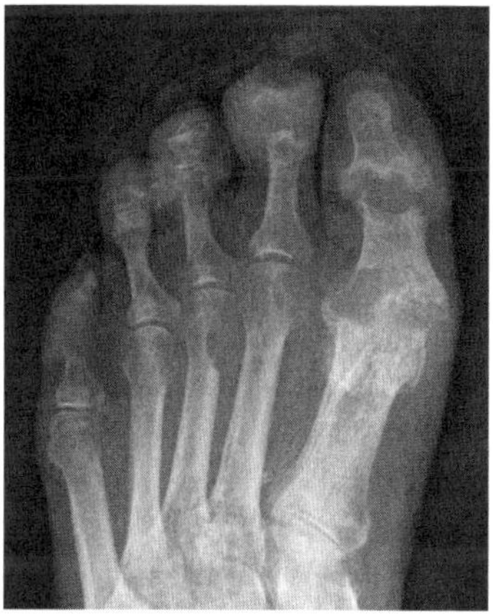

Advanced Imaging Technology

Dopple ultrasonography and magnetic resonance imaging (MRI) can detect inflammation (synovitis) and bone erosions. Dual energy–computed tomography (DECT) can show early signs of the effects of gout on joints, identify tophi, and actually measure the amount of crystal deposits in the affected joint or joints.

Complications from Gout

Untreated gout attacks can become more frequent and last longer, and can cause these serious complications or conditions.

Joint Damage

Hyperuricemia can lead to persistent low-level inflammation between gout attacks, resulting in synovitis, cartilage loss, and bone erosion.

Kidney Stones

Uric acid crystals can develop in the urinary tract and lead to kidney stones (renal calculi) and kidney damage. Kidney stones can cause an infection in the urinary system. People with gout die of kidney disease at four times the rate of people without gout.

Tophi

The formation of tophi is the result of persistent, long-term hyperuricemia in people with gout. See "Chronic Tophaceous Gout," page 14, for more on chronic tophaceous gout.

Other Risks

Because people with gout are at increased risk for metabolic syndrome, they're liable to suffer from the contributing factors of coronary artery disease, hypertension, insulin resistance, and stroke. A study in 2001 showed an association between gout and unhealthy cholesterol and lipid levels. Another study published in the journal *Arthritis & Rheumatism* found that men with gout had an increased risk of heart attacks, even if they had no previous history of heart disease. Other rare complications can occur if gout is left untreated, such as cataracts, dry eye syndrome, and problems with crystal deposits in the lungs.

Treating Your Gout

If you've been diagnosed with gout, your doctor will focus on:

- treating any acute attacks,
- reducing the level of uric acid concentration in your blood to stop the formation of MSU crystals in the joints,
- eliminating already deposited crystals in joints and tophi,
- and treating the disease to prevent future gout flares.

Managing an Acute Attack

The most common procedure used to alleviate the pain of a gout flare-up is a combination of medications and lifestyle recommendations. Anti-inflammatories are used to reduce pain, and a variety of medicines are employed to remove urates or to lower urate levels. Be sure to tell your doctor about all the medicines and vitamins you take, as some of them may elevate your urate levels.

Other things you can do to get relief is elevate the affected joint, avoid bumping or touching it, and apply an ice pack to it for about twenty minutes (but no longer). Be sure to get plenty of bed rest. Your doctor may also decide to remove some fluid from the gouty joint to relieve pain and pressure.

Look over the list of foods that should be avoided, as well as those that are either protective or acceptable (see "A Recommended Diet for Chronic Gout," page 30). Get regular exercise and lose weight if you're overweight.

Medications for an Acute Gout Attack or Flare

The recommended medication for an otherwise healthy adult is a nonsteroidal anti-inflammatory (NSAID). People who can't tolerate NSAIDs are sometimes given corticosteroids or oral colchicine (see below). As with anything that causes pain, a gout flare is best controlled if medications are taken at the first sign of pain or inflammation.

NSAIDs (Nonsteroidal Anti-Inflammatory Drugs)

Over-the-counter NSAIDs include two medicines that most people are familiar with—aspirin and ibuprofen—as well as naproxen and ketoprofen, among others. They should be taken at the maximum anti-inflammatory dose (at least 400 milligrams) in order to be effective. For that reason, people being treated for gout are usually given 400 to 800 milligrams of ibuprofen three to four times a day.

NSAIDs should be taken exactly as prescribed for the shortest time at the lowest dose possible for treatment. Regular use can cause serious health problems, such as heart attack, stroke, and ulcers, and you might also experience allergic reactions and digestive distress. Risks increase if you smoke or drink alcohol or are in poor health (especially if you have heart disease, kidney disease, or liver disease).

If you're allergic to NSAIDs, you may be able to take celecoxib (Celebrex), a COX-2 inhibitor that disrupts the inflammation pathway. Celecoxib and other COX-2 inhibitors are easier on the digestive tract than other NSAIDs. They carry the same risks and warnings, and can cause serious side effects, so be sure to talk to your doctor about these risks. Also alert them to any other drugs you're taking, because celecoxib can have adverse effects if taken with certain other medications and it can alter the effects of other drugs as well.

Colchicine

Colchicine is the classic treatment for gout flares to reduce pain and inflammation, and has been prescribed for hundreds of years. Colchicine is a natural herbal remedy originally isolated from the corm (underground bulb) of the autumn crocus flower (*Colchicum autumnale*). The first recorded use we have of colchicine is by Hippocrates in the fifth century BCE. He used it as a purgative to treat gout but quit using it because of its many adverse effects. The use of colchicine was revived in 1810, but it wasn't until 2009 that nongeneric colchicine with the brand name Colcrys received FDA approval.

It's used less frequently in the United States than elsewhere because of a high incidence of side effects and the fact that it's only successful in relieving symptoms in less than fifty percent of people with gout. Colchicine can also suppress blood cell production and cause nerve and muscular damage in some people, even at a low dose. If your doctor does prescribe colchicine for you, avoid taking it at the same time as grapefruit, because its effects may be altered by grapefruit and cause serious side effects. A number of medications can interact with colchicine and cause side effects as well, so be sure your doctor and pharmacist are aware of all other medicines and supplements you're taking.

Colchicine at a low dose (total of 1.8 mg per day) has been found to be as effective as a high dose (total of 4.8 mg per day). Colchicine at a low dose also has a better safety record.

Corticosteroids

Corticosteroids are strong anti-inflammatory hormones. They bring rapid relief and symptoms usually improve within a few hours of treatment. This type of drug shouldn't be used for long-term treatment, only the shortest time possible. It's reserved for people with severe gout or kidney or liver failure, or who cannot take NSAIDs. If you only have one joint that's affected, the medication might be injected directly into the site; if you have several joints involved, you might receive an oral dose instead.

Don't take a corticosteroid if you have bone marrow disease, diabetes, impaired kidney function, impaired liver function, or heart disease. The list of side effects is diverse, ranging from circulatory problems to wide mood swings. Side effects generally stop when the drug is stopped, but it can be dangerous to stop taking corticosteroids suddenly. Work closely with your doctor if your corticosteroid dosage is reduced.

Treating Chronic Gout

The long-term treatment for gout is to reduce and keep urate levels in body fluids and tissue to a target level of less than 6.8 mg/dL. At this level MSU crystals will no longer form in the body, and MSU crystal deposits will begin to diminish and eventually disappear. This can also reduce and eliminate tophi. Currently, medications are the most effective treatment; diet and other lifestyle measures should be followed to reinforce the medications you might be prescribed.

There are a number of medicines that lower urate levels, referred to as urate-lowering drugs (ULD). Your doctor will start you on a low dose of medication, because too rapid a reduction in urate levels can cause deposits in the joints and surrounding tissues to mobilize and initiate an inflammatory response. If you tolerate a low dose of your medication, your doctor may decide to gradually increase it. Treatment is usually done with a combination of drugs that block urate synthesis by inhibiting xanthine metabolism and agents that promote uric acid excretion.

Urate-lowering therapy (ULT) should not be started during a gout flare. In fact many rheumatologists recommend that ULT not be started until two or three separate gout flares have occurred. However, don't stop your ULT if you experience a flare-up; it should be continued through the flare.

Treatment with ULT is long-term and the medications are expensive. NSAIDs and oral colchicine are also prescribed in small doses for some patients to prevent flares during ULT.

Xanthine Oxidase Inhibitors

This type of drug is effective in reducing urate levels and reversing tophi deposits. Allopurinol was first marketed in 1963 and is one of the most important developments in the treatment of hyperuricemia and gout. It reduces the production of uric acid by blocking the breakdown of hypoxanthine (a purine derivative) to xanthine that then converts to uric acid. Allopurinol can sometimes cause a gout attack when you first take it, so you might be prescribed a NSAID or colchicine for three to six months to counter this.

Febuxostat is an option for people who fail to respond well to or can't tolerate allopurinol. Like allopurinol, febuxostat can cause a gout attack when first administered, so again patients are usually prescribed an NSAID or colchicine for six months to counter this effect.

Both allopurinol and febuxostat can have serious side effects. Check the recommendations that accompany your medication and contact your doctor immediately if you experience any complications. However, a 2014 study published in the journal *Annals of Rheumatic Diseases* showed that allopurinol may reduce the risk of premature death in patients with gout and that the survival benefit may outweigh the risks of these side effects.

Uricosuric Medications and Uricase Replacements

Uricosuric medications increase urate excretion in the urine by blocking urate reabsorption by the kidneys and are used by people who under-excrete uric acid. Sulfinpyrazone, probenecid, and benzbromarone are the most common uricosuric drugs used worldwide. Probenecid (Col-Probenecid) is currently the only uricosuric medication that has FDA approval. Be sure to drink six to eight full glasses of water each day while taking probenecid to prevent kidney stones. Aspirin and other NSAIDs can interfere with uricosuric drugs and can alter their effectiveness, so as with all the other medications prescribed for gout, let your doctor and pharmacist know all the drugs and supplements you take before you start on probenecid.

In order to excrete uric acid efficiently, the enzyme uricase must be present. Uricase converts urate (uric acid) to allantoin, a more easily excreted compound. We lost the ability to synthesize uricase due to a mutation of the uricase gene during human evolution, so we can't effectively remove uric acid from our bodies. Two uricase replacements that are sometimes prescribed are rasburicase (Elitek) and pegloticase (Krystexxa). Rasburicase is used for treating cases of severe gout that don't respond to traditional treatment. It can cause an immune reaction, so sometimes pegloticase is the option chosen. Polyethylene glycol added to pegloticase masks the uricase protein, allowing it to have a longer effect without causing an immune response. Pegloticase is also used by people who can't tolerate allopurinol.

A Recommended Diet for Chronic Gout

Like everyone, people with gout should eat a diet that will help avoid weight gain and includes the recommended nutritional requirements for good health. But there are some important differences. Eliminate or severely limit the consumption of meat and seafood. Instead, eat plant-based sources of protein (beans and vegetables) and plant-based omega-3 fatty acids (walnuts and walnut seed oil, flax seeds and flax seed oil, or hemp seeds and hemp seed oil). Also reduce any foods high in fructose, particularly fruit juices, apples, grapes, and watermelon, and avoid honey and processed foods containing sweetening syrups (corn syrup, agave, molasses, etc.). As was mentioned earlier, reduce alcohol consumption, particularly beer and spirits.

Avoid low-carbohydrate diets that are designed for quick weight loss. When carbohydrate intake is insufficient, your body can't completely burn its own fat. As a consequence, substances called ketones are formed and released into the bloodstream. Ketosis can increase the level of uric acid in your blood.

Foods That Increase Gout Flares

Three groups of food have been shown to be particularly conducive to causing gout flares.

Meat and Seafood

A study cited in the 2005 edition of the *Annals of Internal Medicine* showed that men eating the greatest amount of meat (which is high in purines) had a 41 percent higher risk for gout compared to men eating the least amount of meat. Men eating the most amount of seafood had a 51 percent higher risk of gout than men eating the least amount of seafood. The study showed that consumption of purine-rich vegetables (for example, peas, beans, lentils, spinach, mushrooms, and cauliflower) did not have an increased risk for gout.

The Mayo Clinic gout diet allows for animal protein, but guidelines state to limit the amount consumed to 4 to 6 ounces (113 to 170 grams) a day. The specific language cautions to "avoid or severely limit high-purine foods, such as organ meats, herring, anchovies and mackerel." Be aware that red meat (beef, pork, and lamb) and fatty fish and seafood like tuna, shrimp, lobster, and scallops have all been linked to hyperuricemia and gout. Avoiding purine-rich foods of animal origin will reduce the risk of recurrent gout attacks.

Fructose

In 1993 the *American Journal of Clinical Nutrition* reported on research that indicated a high-fructose diet can cause hyperuricemia in healthy adults. Uric acid levels increase significantly soon after a sugary drink is consumed. Of particular concern are foods and drinks that are high in fructose (fruit juices, fresh fruit) and high-fructose corn syrup (most commercial candy, cakes, and cookies). Dietary recommendations for people with gout suggest avoiding these foods.

The foods with the greatest amounts of fructose are table sugar (sucrose, which is half fructose), high-fructose corn syrup, agave nectar, honey, molasses, maple syrup, and fruit juices. Apple and pear juices in particular contain high levels of fructose. Processed foods that contain these ingredients will also be high in fructose. For people with gout, reducing the consumption of fructose and sugar in general could be as important as the elimination of high-purine foods.

Alcohol

Beer and spirits should be avoided. Wine in moderation is permissible. (See page 18). Drink plenty of water to help flush uric acid from the body.

Foods That Reduce Gout Flares

In a study published in the *New England Journal of Medicine* in 2004, scientists found that consumption of low-fat dairy products reduces the risk of gout in men by half. The reason for this protective effect is not yet known. The consumption of dairy products, even low-fat dairy products, has also been associated with adverse health risks, such as prostate cancer and breast cancer, so their benefits need to be weighed against these risks.

Vegetable protein too seems to have a protective effect, but to a lesser degree. A study cited by the National Institute of Health examining the effects of vitamin C on uric acid suggests that it may be beneficial in the prevention and management of gout. Both regular and decaf coffee also have been reported to have a protective effect in preventing gout flares.

By following the diet and lifestyle guidelines presented here and by your rheumatologist, you'll be able to control how much uric acid your body produces, as well as your ability to eliminate it. These guidelines will also help decrease the number and severity of gout attacks you suffer. But diet alone will not completely control gout. Long-term therapy with urate-lowering medication will be necessary.

Foods to avoid:

- beer
- white bread
- fruit juice and foods containing fructose/sugar
- organ meats
- red meat
- seafood
- yeast-containing foods (breads, yeast spreads)

Foods to eat:

- beans and lentils
- cherries and cherry juice
- coffee
- complex carbohydrates (whole grains, vegetables)
- foods high in vitamin C
- nuts and peanuts
- plant-based omega-3 fatty acids (walnuts, flax seed, hemp seed)
- vegetables, all kinds

Foods that can be consumed in moderation:

- low-fat dairy products
- fruits
- wine

Research for the Future

We're fortunate to live in an age where so much is known about what causes gout and which medications can reduce gout attacks. Out of all the forms of arthritis, gout is perhaps the easiest to control.

The goals now are to make treatments even more effective and possibly preventative. The National Institute of Health has outlined what researchers are focusing on:

1. Doctors are trying to determine which of the current treatments are most effective and at which dosages.
2. A number of new therapies have shown promise in recent studies, including biologic agents that block a chemical called tumor necrosis factor. This chemical is believed to play a role in the inflammation of gout.

3. Research is suggesting that certain foods may actually prevent gout, such as low-fat dairy products and vitamin C.
4. Scientists are also studying the contributions of different types of cells that are involved in both the acute and chronic joint manifestations of gout. They want to better understand how urate crystals activate white blood cells (called neutrophils) and lead to acute gout attacks, affect the immune system and result in chronic gout, and interact with bone cells in a way that causes debilitating bone lesions among people with chronic gout. The hope is that a better understanding of the various inflammatory reactions that occur in gout will provide innovative clues for treatment.
5. Researchers are studying different populations in which gout is prevalent to determine how certain genes and environmental factors may affect blood levels of uric acid.

New Medicines on the Horizon

Several new drugs are being tested as possible highly effective therapies that one day might replace today's standard treatments for gout. Interleukin 1beta (IL-1β) has been identified as a potent agent in the inflammatory process, so suppression of IL-1β is seen as a possible treatment to interrupt the inflammatory process in gout. IL-1βs are effective in people who don't respond well to or can't tolerate other gout medications and are given by injection. Similar drugs being studied are rilonacept, a soluble IL-1 receptor-Fc fusion protein, and canakinumab, an anti–IL-1β antibody. Both have been shown to prevent recurring attacks and are being studied as possible treatments to prevent or treat gout flares.

A number of other therapies have also shown promise in this area, including infliximab (Remicade), an artificial antibody. At present, these medications are very expensive, but hopefully will be more accessible in the future.

Conclusion

Medical science has greatly increased its understanding of gout, but it's still a significant disease and reported cases are increasing worldwide. While we don't know the exact cause of gout and gout cannot be cured, it can be effectively managed with rest, exercise, diet, and medications. Uric acid levels can be reduced, inflammation controlled, gout flares eliminated, and tophi shrunk and completely dissolved.

If you have gouty arthritis, you'll most likely have to take urate-lowering medication for the rest of your life. But with the proper treatment, you can lead a productive life and be free of its crippling effects. Get healthy and manage your gout. All the best to you!

APPENDIX

An Early History of Gout Diagnosis and Treatment

Gout is one of the earliest known diseases, first identified by the Egyptian physician, high priest, and architect Imhotep in 2640 BCE. Much later, Hippocrates, the acknowledged father of western medicine, referenced gout and called it "the unwalkable disease." He described podagra (gout of the foot) and gonagra (gout of the knee) and drew a distinction between it and other types of arthritis.

He treated gout by "administering purgatives either by mouth or by injections; the drinking of asses' milk and whey, and the affusion of cold water to the affected parts, considering that the pain would be alleviated by any application which induced a moderate torpor of the limb." (Garrod 1859, 7) It is interesting that Hippocrates recommended drinking donkey's milk and whey. Recent research has shown that eating low-fat dairy products reduces uric acid levels.

Hippocrates has shown in his five aphorisms on the disease that he had a considerable knowledge of the laws and nature of gout.

The Five Aphorisms of Hippocrates on Gout

VI-28 Eunuchs do not take the gout, nor become bald.

VI-29 A woman does not take the gout, unless her menses be stopped.

VI-30 A youth does not get gout before sexual intercourse.

VI-40 In gouty affections, inflammation subsides within forty days.

XI-55 Gouty affections become active in spring and in autumn.

From earliest times, gout has been thought to be a disease of an indulgent, intemperate lifestyle. Pliny, in the reign of Nero during the first century CE, commented on the prevalence of gout, saying it was "almost unknown in the early, more virile days of the Empire." He called out the Roman population for living a life of luxury and sloth seeing the disease as yet "another harbinger of impending decadence, clearly attributable to riotous living and debauchery." (Llewellyn 1921, 2)

Seneca, also in the first century CE, observes, "The nature of women is not altered but their manner of living, for while they rival the men in every kind of licentiousness, they equal them too in their very bodily disorders. Why need we then be surprised at seeing so many of the female sex afflicted with gout." (Llewellyn 1921, 5)

Galen Aelius Galenus (CE129–200/217), better known as Galen of Pergamon, attributed gout to intemperance, debauchery, and heredity. He wrote, "In the time of Hippocrates there were only a few who suffered from podagra, such was the moderation in living, but in our own times, when sensuality has touched the highest conceivable point, the number of patients with the gout has grown to an extent that cannot be estimated." (Llewellyn 1921, 2) He was the first to describe tophi.

From Aretaeus of Cappadocia in the second century CE we get: "The reluctance which the victims display to assigning the malady to its true cause—their own excesses—preferring to attribute it to a new shoe, a long walk, or an injury. But, for the true nature of the disease, he, with humility and piety, avows that its secret origin is known only to the gods." Aretaeus thought that a predisposition for gout could be inherited. (Llewellyn 1921, 5)

Caelius Aurelianus, a Greco-Roman physician of the fifth century CE, also looked upon gout as a hereditary disease and considered that indigestion, intemperance, cold, debauchery, and injuries were the principle causes. He was of the opinion that the disease was located in the tendons and ligaments. He recommended an abstemious diet and regular exercise in the treatment of gout, recommendations that are today given to patients.

In the sixth century CE, the Byzantine Christian physician Alexander of Tralles first recorded colchicine as a specific treatment for gout.

"In the middle or latter half of the thirteenth century, Demetrius Pepagomenos wrote a treatise on gout. He wrote, the 'predisposing causes are said to be excess of food and wine, indolence, indigestion, retention of natural excretions, and debilitating causes, as over-exercise and fatigue and too great indulgence in venery.'" (Adams 1886, 17–18)

In 1679 Anton Leeuwenhoek first described the substance in gouty tophi as crystals, and in 1797 Wollaston identified these as monosodium urate (MSU) crystals, which he took from a tophus on his own ear.

"According to Mason Good 'Gout is one of the maladies which seem to have been common in England in its earliest ages of barbarism. It is frequently noticed by Anglo-Saxon historians and the name assigned to it is *Fot-adl.*'"(Llewellyn 1921, 3)

Its prevalence should come as no surprise considering the lifestyle of the privileged at the time—grand feasts with meats, sweets, and rich foods of all kinds washed down with copious amounts of ale.

During the seventeenth and eighteenth centuries, gout was thought a mark of high social status and a blessing. It was believed gout offered protection from other diseases and it prolonged life. People actually went so far as to try to bring on a gout flare-up by overindulging in rich food and alcoholic drink.

As noted, Aretaeus (second century) and Aurelianus (fifth century) both thought that gout could be inherited, but it was not until the eighteenth century that a Scottish physician named William Cullen proposed a genetic connection and William Scheele idendified uric acid.

In 1859 Sir Albert Barring Garrod showed that gout was strongly associated with hyperuricemia and recommended a low-purine diet to treat gout patients. At the end of the nineteenth century, Haig showed that limiting the consumption of purine-rich food could reduce uric acid levels.

In 1931 Garrod's son, Sir Archibald Garrod, proposed that gout should be classified as an inborn metabolic disorder. Somewhat later, diagnosis of gout by detection of monosodium urate (MSU) crystals in joint fluid with polarizing light miscroscopy was first done.

In the 1960s two gout researchers, J. S. Faries and D. J. MacCarty conducted an experiment with themselves as the subjects. They injected their left knees with 20 milligrams of (MSU) crystals each. They quickly developed an acute inflammation reaction with all the symptoms of an acute gouty attack. Four hours later they were still prostrate and suffering from intense pain in the affected knee. This experiment established the fact that MSU crystals are indeed the initial triggers of a gout flare-up.

Colchicine had been the classic drug to treat gout flares for centuries, but it fell out of favor because of the risks and side effects associated with its use. It came back into use in modern times around 1810, but it has again fallen out of favor. In 2009 the FDA approved a nongeneric colchicine with the brand name Colcrys.

By the 1940s acute gout was being treated with aspirin. In 1951 probenecid was developed to lower uric acid levels, and in 1963 allopurinol was also approved by the FDA to lower uric acid levels. Allopurinol quickly became the drug of choice to treat hyperuricemia.

GLOSSARY

From the National Institute of Health

Corticosteroids

Powerful anti-inflammatory hormones made naturally in the body or man-made for use as medicine are known as corticosteroids. Injections of corticosteroid drugs are sometimes used to treat inflammation in the shoulder, knee, and other joints.

Diuretics

Diuretics are a type of medication that promotes the formation and output of urine. They are prescribed to treat the accumulation of excess fluid in bodily tissues that can result from diseases of the kidneys, liver, lungs, or heart. They may also be used to treat high blood pressure or glaucoma, a condition in which pressure builds up inside the eye.

DNA

Deoxyribonucleic acid, known as DNA, is a self-replicating material present in nearly all living organisms as the main constituent of chromosomes. It is the carrier of genetic information.

Hyperuricemia

The presence of elevated levels of uric acid (urate) in the blood is called hyperuricemia.

NSAIDs

Nonsteroidal anti-inflammatory drugs, or NDAIDs, are a class of medications, available over the counter or with a prescription, that ease pain and inflammation.

Podagra

Gout in the big toe is called podagra.

Pseudogout

Pseudogout is a condition often mistaken for gout that results from the deposit of calcium phosphate crystals (not uric acid crystals as in gout) in the joints and other tissues. This condition is also called chondrocalcinosis.

Purines

Purines are nitrogen-containing compounds that come from the cells within the body (endogenous), or from outside of the body, from the foods we eat (exogenous). Purines are part of the DNA and RNA within the nuclei of cells all animal and plant cells and are more concentrated in certain high protean foods. Purines break down into uric acid.

RNA

Ribonucleic acid (RNA) is a nucleic acid present in all living cells. Its principal role is to act as a messenger carrying instructions from DNA for controlling the synthesis of proteins, although in some viruses RNA rather than DNA carries the genetic information.

sUA

For the long-term treatment of gout, target levels for sUA (serum uric acid) should be < 6.0 mg/dL.

Synovial fluid.

The slippery fluid produced by the synovium (joint lining) to lubricate the joints is called synovial fluid.

Tophi

Tophi are nodular masses of uric acid crystals that sometimes form in the soft tissue of people with chronic gout. Although tophi are most common around the fingers, elbows, and big toe, they can occur in virtually any part of the body. (The singular is tophus.)

Uric acid

Uric acid is a substance that results from the breakdown of purines, which are part of all human tissue and are found in many foods.

REFERENCES

Abeles, AM, Pillinger, M. New therapeutic options for gout here and on the horizon. 2010. www.musculoskeletalnetwork.com/gout/content/article/1145622/1533314

Adams F, editor. *The Genuine Works of Hippocrates. I and II.* New York: Wood, 1886.

Al-Ashkar, F. Gout and pseudogout. *Cleveland Clinic Journal of Medicine.* www.clevelandclinicmeded.com/medicalpubs/diseasemanagement/rheumatology/gout-and-pseudogout/

American College of Rheumatology (ACR). www.rheumatology.org/

Choi HK, Mount DB, Reginato AM. Pathogenesis of gout. *Ann Intern Med.* 2005; 143:499–516.

Choi, HK, Atkinson, K, Karlson, EW, Willett, W, Curhan. G. 2004. Purine-rich foods, dairy and protein intake, and the risk of gout in men. *N Engl J Med.* 2004; 350:1093–1103.

Choi, HK, Curhan, G. Soft drinks, fructose consumption, and the risk of gout in men: prospective cohort study. *BMJ* 2008; 336 doi: http://dx.doi.org/10.1136/bmj.39449.819271.BE

Garrod, AB. *The Nature and Treatment of Gout and Rheumatic Gout,* London: Walton and Maberly, 1859.

Rheumatology Network Staff. Higher gout prevalence with growth in obesity and hypertension. *The Journal of Musculoskeletal Medicine.* Vol. 28, No. 9. (2011) www.musculoskeletalnetwork.com/gout/content/article/1145622/1942726.

Krishnan, E, Lingala, B, and Bhalla, V. Low levels of lead in the blood and the occurrence of gout. *Ann Inten Med.* Vol, 157, 233–241. (2012) http://annals.org/article.aspx?articleid=1351359

Llewellyn, J. *Gout.* St. Louis: CV Mosby Company, 1921

Martinon, Fabio. Mechanisms of uric acid crystal-mediated autoinflammation. Immunological Reviews. Vol. 233: 218-232 (2010)

Mayo Clinic Staff, Mayo Clinic. Gout diet: what's allowed, what's not. www.mayoclinic.com/health/gout-diet/MY01137

Medication Guide Colcrys, URL Pharma Inc, revised December 2009.

Medication Guide Allopurinol, Watson Pharma Private Limited, revised March 2009. 184001, 03098.

Medication Guide Celebrex, G.D. Searle LLC, Division of Pfizer Inc, New York, New York, June 2009.

Medication Guide ULORIC, Takeda Pharmaceuticals America, Inc., 2009, 2011, ULR015 R2.

National Institute of Health. www.niams.nih.gov/Health_Info/Gout/default.asp#do

Sandy, JS. A Phase II Multidose Study of Intravenous PEG-uricase in patients with refractory gout. www.clinicaltrials.gov/ct2/show/NCT00111657

Sivera F, et al. *Annals of Rheumatic Disease* The EULAR Journal *Ann Rheum Dis* 2013;1-8. Doi:10.1136/annrheumdis-2013-203325, 3E Recommendations in Rheumatology. 3e (Evidence, Expertise, Exchange) Initiative. Published on line: http://ard.bmj.com/content/early/2013/07/17/annrheumdis-2013-203325.full

Sydenham, T, Wallis, G. 1788. *A Treatise of the Gout and Dropsy*. London: N.p.

ABOUT THE AUTHOR

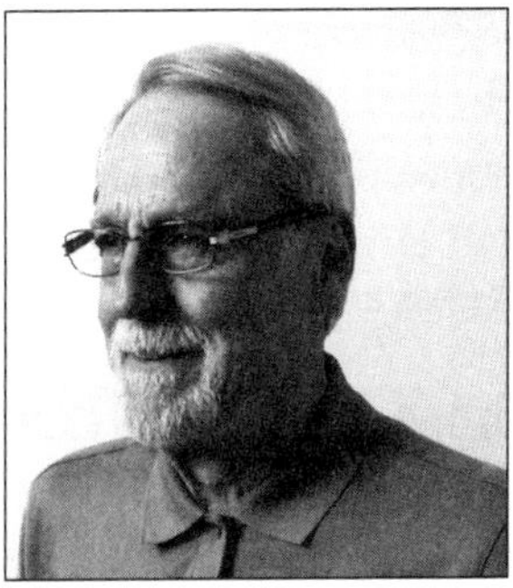

Warren Jefferson works as a graphic artist, photographer, and research writer for the Book Publishing Company, which publishes books on vegan and raw foods lifestyles, alternative health, and Native American culture. He has edited and worked on numerous publications on a variety of subjects.

His first health book, *The Neti Pot for Better Health*, gives readers the information needed to use this traditional personal health tool to combat the flu and to relieve allergies and sinus problems. His second health book, *Colloidal Silver Today*, offers the latest findings and research on the low-tech alternative germ killer colloidal silver. It includes instructions for building a low-cost generator to produce colloidal silver at home for pennies an ounce.

Warren and his wife Barbara have four children and five grandchildren. They are founding members of an intentional community in Tennessee, called The Farm, which is dedicated to promoting sustainable living, natural childbirth, and nonviolence. He is active in the local community and works with the Victim Offender Reconciliation Program as a certified mediator helping people resolve conflicts and differences without going to court.